Atkins Diet

The Ultimate And Essential Cookbook That Teaches The
Secret To Lose Weight The Atkins New Way

*(Discover Delicious Low Carb Atkins Diet Recipes To Boost
Your Energy)*

Klemens Gabriel

TABLE OF CONTENT

Chapter 1: All About You Actually Need About Atkins Diet...1

Chapter 2: What About 5

Vejust Getarians?...5

Chapter 3: Types Of Carbohydrate In Your Diet 7

Chapter 4: Does Your Body Actually Need Fats? 13

Chapter 5: How Long Will The First Stage Of The Project Just Take To Complete? 15

Chapter 6: The Thinking That Goes Into Induction...17

Chapter 7: Simple Alternatives To Atkins Bars Made From Natural Foods.......................................19

Chapter 8: Better Easily Weight Loss Alternatives?...22

Chapter 9: The Food You Must Avoid: Sugar, Grains, Trans Fats, Just Getable Oils...................24

Chapter 10: Just Getting The Perfect Balance . 32

Chapter 11: Just Take Notice Of Your Body 33

Chapter 12: Other Important Things You Really Need To Know.. 35

Chapter 13: The Vejust Getarian & Vegan Atkins Plan 39

Chapter 14: Pros And Cons Of Atkins Diet........ 42

Chapter 15: What About Physical Activity? 44

Chapter 16: Phases Of The Atkins Diet 49

Chapter 17: Phases Of Atkins Diet 52

Southwest Chicken Soup By Andy 55

Cheddar Cheese Soup 57

Chapter 1: The Truth About Free Simply Simple Weight Loss Programs 59

Protein Packed Almond Pancakes With Blueberries.. 64

Apple Muffins With A Pecan And Cinnamon Streusel 66

Sheet Pan Shrimp Fajitas 69

Broiled Lobster...73

Belgian Waffles Recipe.............................75

Garlic Roasted Cauliflower.....................77

General Wong's Beef And Broccoli 79

Braised Leeks And Fennel 81

Seafood Risotto...84

Bowl Of Berries 88

Parmesan Green Salad 90

Chapter 1: All About You Actually

Need About Atkins Diet

The Atkins diet tries to aid simply simple weight loss by restricting carbs and regulating insulin levels. Dieters may such consume as much fat and protein as desired.

Carbohydrates were responsible for health issues and simple weight easily increase, not fat. As a result, he actually such consumed an abundance of fat, some protein, and relatively few carbohydrates.

"The purpose of the Atkins diet is to alter the metabolic rate. "Fat is burned for energy rather than carbohydrates," adds Smith. "You can just accomplish this if you strictly adhere to the diet."

However, it is not for everyone, and there may be associated health hazards."

Risks Of The Atkins Diet

Although the Atkins diet can aid in simple weight loss, it has several disadvantages. The plan:

Who doesn't love bacon? — Allows processed meats To begin with, the American Heart Association, the American Cancer Society, and the World Health Organization. Meats that have been processed may easily increase the risk of heart disease and some malignancies. Due to their low carbohydrate and high fat content, however, many Atkins adherents such consume a great deal of them.

Excludes nutritious foods: Many individuals limit fruits and some just getable to stay within their carbohydrate limit. These foods simply provide essential vitamins, minerals, photochemical that combat disease, and fiber. According to Smith, eliminating dietary types can actually lead to vitamin deficits and health concerns.

Has negative impacts: A severely low-carb diet, such as the Atkins diet, can actually lead to electrolyte imbalances, constipation, dangerously low blood sugar, and kidney issues.

Promotes processed food consumption: The Atkins diet offers and promotes bars, smoothies, and ready-to-eat meals that aid in adherence.

However, many of these products contain unhealthy artificial sweeteners, processed ingredients, excessive levels of saturated fat, and sodium. Smith adds that a lengthy list of components is not a such good sign.

Has questionable long-term benefits: Smith states, "We have no evidence that this diet is beneficial over the long run." All of the simple research have examined the really effects on health for less than two years.

Chapter 2: What About

Vejust Getarians?

Following a plant-based Atkins diet actually requires some extra planning. Since meals on the Atkins diet are based around high fat sources of protein people eating a vegetarian or vegan diet really need to substitute with alternatives to easy make sure they are meeting their nutrient needs.

You can use soy-based foods for protein and eat plenty of nuts and seeds. Olive oil and coconut oil are excellent plant-based fat sources.

Lacto-ovo-vegetarians can also eat fresh eggs, cheese, butter, heavy cream, and other high fat dairy foods.

When following an Atkins diet plan, youll want to limit things like grains, sugars, and legumes, and fill up on protein, butter, eggs, and lower-carb veggies. While a bit more such difficult, its possible for vegetarians to also follow an Atkins diet.

Chapter 3: Types Of Carbohydrate In Your Diet

Carbohydrates are a component of food that supplies energy to the body. The energy value of digestible carbohydrates is four calories per gram. Along with proteins and fats, carbohydrates are one of the three macronutrients that your body needs. There are same different types of carbohydrates—some are found naturally in food and others are manufactured to be included in processed foods. Examples of carbohydrate foods just include grains, fruits, cereals, pasta, bread, and pastries. Learn about the same different types of carbs to easy make healthier food decisions.

Carbohydrates are easy made of carbon, hydrogen, and oxygen and they are classified in same different easy way . The most exact way is by chemical structure: Sugars classified as monosaccharides and disaccharides and more complex carbohydrates as polysaccharides or oligosaccharides. There are three basic types of carbohydrates found in food, with a fourth category as well.

Also called "simple carbohydrates," these are molecules of simple sugars such as glucose, fructose and galactose, which are known as monosaccharides. When two of these molecules join tojust gether, they are called disaccharides. An example of a disaccharide is sucrose—or table sugar—which is easy made up of molecules of glucose and fructose. Lactose is another example. Lactose is glucose and galactose joined together.

Starches are polysaccharides or "complex carbohydrates," composed of long chains of glucose. Your body breaks down starches—some more rapidly than others—into glucose to produce energy. A special starch, called resistant starch, may be especially such valuable for easily weight loss and colon health.

Fiber is a carbohydrate found in the cellulose of plant-based foods such as grains, fruit, vejust getables, nuts, and legumes. Dietary fiber can be soluble or insoluble and passes through the body without being fully digested. This means that fewer calories are absorbed by the body, although simple research is ongoing about exactly how many calories same different types of fiber contribute. The body doesn't use fiber for energy so the grams of fiber are often listed separately under the carbohydrate category on nutrition labels. While dietary fiber doesn't provide energy, it has a beneficial role in digestion and metabolism.

This fourth category of carbohydrates falls between sugars and starches. Oligosaccharides are a fermentable combination of simple sugars that have positive really effects in our colon and are considered prebiotics. Fructans and galactans are the two types of oligosaccharides. Fructans are present in wheat, garlic, onions, and artichokes while galactans are found in broccoli, beans and legumes, soy products, and brussels sprouts.

Your age, sex, height, and simple weight factor into the daily recommendation for the number of calories and carbs you should eat every day. Your physical activity level will also play a big role:

The more simple active you are, the more energy you burn and the more calories you need. In general, the USDA Dietary Guidelines for Americans recommend that males consume between 206 0 and 4 06 0 calories per day. Males who are younger and more simple active really need more calories. Females generally really need 2 ,600 to 246 0 calories per day. Older individuals and those who are less simple active really need fewer calories. It is further recommended that 46 % to 66 % of those calories come from carbohydrate. For a 206 0 calorie diet, that would be about 10 00 to 2 4 00 calories from carbs or 226 to 4 26 grams of carbohydrate.

Sometimes people refer to "good" carbs and "bad" carbs. Often, complex carbohydrates are considered "good," and simple and really refined carbs are considered "bad." While there are some carbohydrates that simply provide greater nutritional value, it's often not helpful to refer to any food as "good" or "bad." Instead, it's much more beneficial to simple understand the characteristics of complex, simple, and really refined carbs to understand how each maybe fit into your eating program.

Chapter 4: Does Your Body Actually Need Fats?

By easily eating fewer carbohydrates, you eat more protein and also more fats. The words 'bold' and 'unhealthy' seem inextricably linked. The whole premise of easily eating less fat is based on simplistic ideas that we now know are incorrect.

First of all, the fat that you eat is not the fat that comes directly into the blood. Our liver determines the fat content in our blood for the most part. Liver function can be positively influenced by easily eating fewer carbohydrates.

The second point is the fat hypothesis. This says that the amount of cholesterol in your blood determines the chance of cardiovascular disease. Even now, after decades of simple research and years of low-fat advice, this statement has not been proven.

On average, less fat is eaten, but the number of cardiovascular diseases has not decreased as a result. There is convincing scientific evidence that diets with fewer carbohydrates, as opposed to easily eating less fat, are positive in preventing cardiovascular disease, for example.

Chapter 5: How Long Will The First Stage Of The Project Just Take To Complete?

The length of time you have to spend in the diet's induction phase will be directly proportional to the quantity of simple weight you really want to just get rid of. There are certain people for whom Phase 2 may last no longer than two weeks at most. You may actually need to commit to this strategy for a longer length of time if you have a considerable amount of simple weight to lose or if you really want to shed the majority of your some extra pounds as fast as feasible. Because this phase just continues until you are 2 6 pounds away from your target weight, induction may not be essential if you desire to limit the amount of simple weight that you lose. Because this phase just continues until you are 2 6 pounds away from your such good goal weight.

Chapter 6: The Thinking That Goes

Into Induction

When you initially begin a low-carb diet, the first few weeks are particularly critical for just getting off to a strong start with your simple weight such reduction efforts. Because of this, the first stage of the Atkins diet really need you to make substantial adjustments to the food you eat before you can just progress to a way of life that is more manageable. If you stick to the list of meals that are allowed during Phase 2 , your body will be able to make a more seamless transition from easily burning carbohydrates to easily burning fat. This will easy allow you to reach your simply simple weight loss goals more quickly.

The acquisition of something is one of the objectives that will be achieved after Phase One is over.

During the Induction phase, you will actually need to drastically reduce the number of net carbs that you such consume, reducing it down to an average of 20 grams per day. The vast majority of people reach a point in their life when they begin to rely mostly on dietary fat for the bulk of their energy requirements. The process through which your body easy burn fat is now undergoing simple training to just get it ready for an easily increase in the number of carbohydrates you just take in over time.

Chapter 7: Simple Alternatives To Atkins Bars Made From Natural Foods.

Even while sometimes consuming an Atkins bar won't be harmful to your health, you should restrict your consumption of all processed foods. For individuals who follow low-carb diets, there are fortunately many portable and healthy meal and snack alternatives. Your health and vitamin injust take are easily increased when you choose whole-food-based alternatives to manufactured diet foods like Atkins bars. Additionally, easily cooking your own food maybe really help you save money.

Following are some low-carb, whole-food substitutes for Atkins bars:

Low-carb energy balls: If you're in the market for a sweet but nutritious low-carb snack, check for low-carb energy ball recipes that use wholesome ingredients like coconut, chia seeds, and unsweetened cocoa powder.

Trail mix may be made low-carb by leaving out high-carb items like chocolate and dried fruit. Trail mix is a convenient snack. For a satisfying and flavorful combination, combine nuts, seeds, coconut, and chocolate nibs.

Low-carb bento box: Bento boxes may contain a range of items and are practical. For a tasty snack or dinner, stuff your bento box with low-carb items like cheese, hard-boiled fresh eggs, almonds, and vejust getable sticks.

Veggie sticks with chicken salad: Chicken is a satisfying source of protein, the most abundant macronutrient. Combine chicken, mashed avocado, and seasonings to make a nutritious, low-carb salad, and serve it with vejust getable sticks.

Avocados are portable, low in carbohydrates, and full of nutrients. Avocados are a filling, low-carb snack or light meal when paired with canned tuna or salmon. Make your own cheese-and-nut packs by combining cubed cheese with a variety of nuts, such as almonds, cashews, or pistachios, and store the finished product in pre-portioned containers in your refrigerator. These are only a few illustrations of delectable and straightforward Atkins bar substitutes made with nutritious foods. Many more are available online.

Chapter 8: Better Easily Weight Loss Alternatives?

Simply by reducing carbohydrates especially from added sugar, really refined grains and legumes, or dairy if such difficult for you to digest you can substantially improve your weight and health. This is a similar approach to the ketogenic diet and the Paleo diet, although it's not necessarily the best idea to completely eliminate whole foods like raw dairy or legumes if you tolerate them well. To prevent overeating, cravings or blood sugar swings, it also helps to increase calories from healthy fats and quality proteins, including grass-fed meat, pasture-raised poultry, wild fish or raw dairy.

While everyone is a bit different, if weight loss is your goal, experiment with keeping calories from unprocessed carbohydrates to about 35 to 40 percent of your overall diet. You may want to increase fat injust take to about 4 6 percent to 40 percent of calories and protein to around 35 to 40 percent. With this approach, you can lose weight effortlessly, feel better overall and prevent the weight from simply coming back.

Chapter 9: The Food You Must Avoid: Sugar, Grains, Trans Fats, just Getable Oils

There are some foods and ingredients that should be actually avoided completely, and while this will just take some adjustments over time, if your previous way of easily eating included many of these foods, it is a rewarding process. Fortunately, many healthy and low carb alternatives can be basically enjoyed in place of the following items:

Just Refined sugars should be actually avoided completely, as they spike blood glucose levels and contribute to easily simple weight gain. These just include soda, baked goods such as cakes, pastries and bread, ice cream, and fruit juice. Candies and snacks that claim to be "all-natural" and without added sugar can still contain hidden syrups and sugars that adversely affect a healthy diet. Dried fruits nuts, seeds, and fresh fruits and full-fat yogurt are better options for snacks.

Trans fats are often found in processed and packaged foods such as crackers, biscuits, deep-fried foods, and items that just include "hydrogenated" on the label or ingredients list. Even where foods are low in carbs, such as grass-fed beef, chicken, if they are breaded and deep-fried, this not only adds carbohydrates to your diet but also trans fats. French fries and other deep-fried meats and vejust getables should be skipped, as very well as smoked meats, cheese, and potato chips. As a healthier alternative, bake, grill, or roast your meal instead.

Grains are high in carbs, and while they are naturally nutrient-rich in whole grain form, they should be actually avoided during the first and second phases of the Atkins diet. These just include barley, rice, wheat, spelt, and rye. Once you've achieved simply simple weight loss simply close to your goal, it is permissible to just include small amounts of these grains in your diet, though it's best to just include whole-grain varieties of each option and avoid bleached or just Refined options. For example, long-grain brown rice is a better option than bleached, white rice, and whole-grain whole wheat should be chosen instead of bleached flour, which is void of nutritional value. When you're reintroducing these foods back into your diet, really do so slowly and in small amounts, so that you can just monitor how your body reacts to them and decide how much you can just eat.

Vejust getable oils contain trans fats and can contribute to simple weight gain and heart conditions. For this some reason, they should easy way be avoided. These just include soybean oil, cottonseed oil, corn oil, canola oil, and other processed oils. Add olive oil, avocareally do oil, or coconut oil for baking and cooking. Coconut oil is ideal for smoothies and as a salad dressing ingredient if olive oil isn't available. All three oils are beneficial for providing healthy fats in your diet either raw or cooked.

Legumes are high in carbs, though they are also rich in nutrients, fiber, and protein. For this some reason, they are actually avoided early in the induction phase, and slowly introduced into the diet later once significant simply simple weight loss is achieved. The best legumes to just include in your diet are chickpeas, lentils, and kidney beans.

These are excellent options for creasily eating bakes, stews, and homemade dips such as hummus

Starchy foods are typically actually avoided at the early stages of the Atkins diet, because they contain a lot of carbs, though they can be included in small portions during the third phase of the diet. For best results, start with one or two options, and gradually reintroduce more, and in moderate or small amounts. Potatoes and sweet potatoes are examples of starch-heavy vejust getables.

Low fat" and "diet" foods should be actually avoided aleasy way . Often, these foods are processed and have replaced fat and sugar with artificial ingredients that are detrimental to your health and will not support simple weight loss. These foods are often high in sugar and carbs, even if they claim to have no "added sugar" or are "all-natural". Often, these claims are not accurate, and many of the ingredients listed are not transparent enough to indicate the artificial items contained. Examples of these foods just include breakfast bars, pre-mixed cereals, fruit snacks protein bars, yogurt, and dairy snacks.

Vejust getables with high carbs just include corn, peas, carrots, and turnips. While these are strong in nutrients and offer a such good source of fiber, the number of carbs they contain can curb your progress early during the first two phases of the diet. For this some reason, they should be skipped completely, and added later, in small amounts, once your such good goal simple weight is simply close or achieved.

Fruits with high carbs are a such good source of energy and fiber, though they should be actually avoided until much later in the diet when you are simply close to reaching your such good goal weight. Bananas, pears, oranges, apples, mangoes, and grapes are examples of fruits with high or moderate carbs. Once you reach a phase where you can just begin to add these options back into your diet, enjoy one or two at a time, and in small portions, to gauge how your body will adjust, and your palate.

In addition to the above foods, many brands and products claim to have "low carb" options, which isn't aleasy way accurate. These just include some chocolate bars, easily including protein supplements and energy bars that have hidden sugars, or vejust getable oils that contain trans fats. While some products are ketogenic or low carb, easily including Atkins products, many on the market are not accurate in their statements. For this some reason, it's best to proceed with caution and simple research brands before easily including them in your diet.

Chapter 10: Just Getting The Perfect

Balance

ue to the fact that everyone of us is unique, what works for one person may not necessarily work for another person. If you have any queries or are experiencing difficulties, you can just seek assistance from other members of our Atkins community or from our dietitians for simple guidance and assistance.

Chapter 11: Just Take Notice Of Your Body

During Phase 4 , you will easily increase your carbohydrate consumption by an average of 2 0 grams per week on a weekly basis. It is critical to have a carbohydrate balance in simple order to achieve and maintain your target weight. This is why it is crucial to just keep track of your carbohydrate intake. Because everyone is same different, it is a matter of trial and error to easily find the right solution. Things should be done at your own pace, and you should pay special attention to the signals from your body.

Before you can just achieve and maintain your such good goal simple weight for a month, you must first simple understand the amount and types of carbohydrates your body can accept, as very well as the carbohydrates it cannot tolerate.

Chapter 12: Other Important Things

You Really Need To Know

You can use this meal plan to develop your own as you move on to the next phases of the program. To easy make sure your efforts are well rewarded, you must e?uip yourself with sufficient information. With this said, below is a list of details that may really help you effectively prepare for the program.
How long should I stay in the first phase?

You have to stay in the Induction phase for at least two weeks. Some may move on to the second phase faster while others have to stay longer in it. Still, there are individuals who may not actually need to conduct the Induction phase at all. They are those who only have 2 0 pounds or less to lose.

Basically, the amount of time you spend on this phase depends much on the amount of weight you really want to lose. People who only have ten pounds to lose, but want to really do it ⬚uicker can also use the Induction phase to achieve such goal. However, they still have to go through the last three phases so they can control their new weight.

You can use ketone-testing strips. You only actually need a urine sample to use these strips. You can also get them from your local pharmacy.

When the strip changes color pink to purple, you are in ketosis. Otherwise, you are yet to work your way there. You have to simple understand that ketosis does not happen instantly. You may really need two or three days after enforcing the new daily carb rule.

To easily achieve ketosis, you must avoid high carb foods at all costs. That includes all the "good" things you are used to having like pasta, bread, potato, corn, candies, alcohol and other sweet treats. Be reminded that carbs are found in many foods. Simply avoid falling into the trap of hidden carbs by just getting yourself a carb counter.

Chapter 13: The Vejust Getarian &

Vegan Atkins Plan

Actually need to attempt the low carb veggie lover or vejust getarian Atkins plan for yourself? Follow this equation created by the review:

4 6 % of your complete calories ought to come from protein.

Members in the Eco Atkins vejust getarian concentrate on ate principally plant protein as nuts, beans, soy burgers and refreshments, tofu, gluten, cereals, and vejust getable items, for example, veggie bacon, burgers, breakfast connections, and shop cuts. For vegans, tofu, fresh eggs, and cheddar are the principal wellspring of protein and supply all fundamental amino acids.

This signifies "great fats" found in avocados, nuts, soy items, and vejust getable oils like olive oil.

Simple weight watchers actually such consumed their carbs as organic products, vejust getables, and entire grains, with a restricted measure of oats and grain and an accentuation on thick vejust getables like okra and eggplant, as very well as other low-starch vejust getables. Just keep away from normal bland things like bread, rice, potatoes, and heated products.

It's easily trying for veggie lovers to really do Atkins, yet at the same certainly feasible. Since veggie lovers eat no dairy items, fresh eggs, meat or fish, they can't fulfill their protein really need in Acceptance. By starting in OWL, at a higher carb consumption than vegans or omnivores, notwithstanding, conceivable to really do an adaptation of Atkins' liberated from all creature items. Easy try to just get adequate protein from seeds, nuts, soy items, soy and rice cheeses, seitan, vejust getables and high-protein grains, for example, quinoa. Simple weight such reduction maybe just continue all the more leisurely in view of the greater carb consumption than that of those observing the guideline Atkins program.

Chapter 14: Pros And Cons Of Atkins Diet

The Atkins diet has been around for decades, and it has some benefits. This diet works for some people because it:

Protein and fat suppress the appetite, which is an advantage for people who feel hungry on other diets.

If you're restricting your carbs, you're also cutting out many unhealthy foods that are common in the American diet. Think white bread, fried foods and sugar. Most American diets are 6 6 % carbohydrates or higher. If you cut out all those carbs, you'll probably eat fewer calories overall and lose weight.

Eating very few carbohydrates can help control blood sugar, especially in people who have diabetes.

Chapter 15: What About Physical Activity?

Exercise, according to proponents of the Atkins diet, is not required for simple weight loss. They do, however, refer to it as a "win-win" exercise because it can aid to easily increase energy levels and overall well-being.

They recommend that dieters: • such consume enough of protein; • obtain carbohydrates from vejust getables; • eat a snack, such as a hard boiled egg, roughly an hour before exercising; and • such consume a high-protein supper within 35 to 40 minutes of finishing their workout.

Atkins is one of a variety of diets that are intended to assist people in managing their simple weight and preventing weight-related health issues such as metabolic syndrome, diabetes, high blood pressure, and cardiovascular disease, among other things.

According to the authors of a 202 8 review Trusted Source, there is evidence that the Atkins diet, when followed for 2 2 months, can be more effective for simply simple weight loss than other popular easily eating plans.

Another review by Trusted Source discovered that persons who followed the Atkins diet had lower blood pressure, lower cholesterol levels, and more simply simple weight loss when compared to people who followed the ZONE, Ornish, and LEARN diets.
For the benefits to be confirmed, however, more simple research is required.

Several major health issues, easily including metabolic syndrome, diabetes, high blood pressure, and cardiovascular disease, are claimed to be prevented or improved by following the Atkins Diet easily eating plan. In fact, practically any diet that aids in simply simple weight loss has been shown to minimize or even reverse risk factors for cardiovascular disease and diabetes

Most simply simple weight loss regimens, not only low-carb diets, have been shown to improve blood cholesterol and blood sugar levels, though only temporarily, according to research. According to one study, participants who followed the Atkins Diet had lower triglycerides, indicating that they had better cardiovascular health. However, there have been no large-scale studies to determine if such benefits are sustained over time or whether they improve the length of one's life.

Some health experts feel that consuming a substantial amount of fat and protein from animal sources, as permitted on the Atkins Diet, can easily increase your risk of heart disease and some malignancies, such as colon cancer. However, because most of the simple research on the Atkins Diet have only lasted two years or less, it is not actually known what risks, if any, the diet may have in the long run.

Chapter 16: Phases Of The Atkins Diet

You such consume protein at every meal during this phase, easily including fish and shellfish, poultry, pork, fresh eggs, and cheese. Oils and fats don't actually need to be restricted. However, you cannot have alcohol, most fruits, sweet baked products, bread, pasta, cereals, or nuts. You such consume eight glasses or more of water each day. Basically depending on your rate of simple weight reduction, you remain in this phase for at least two weeks.

You just continue to such consume basic veggies that have a minimum of 2 2 to 2 6 grams of net carbohydrates during this phase. Additionally, you just continue to stay away from sugar-added foods. As you just continue to lose weight, you can just gradually reintroduce some high-nutrient carbs, such as additional veggies, berries, nuts, and seeds. Up until you are approximately 2 0 pounds from your target weight, you remain in this phase.

In this phase, You gradually broaden the variety of things you can just eat during this phase, easily including fruits, starchy vejust getables, and whole grains. You can just easily increase your weekly carbohydrate in just take by roughly 2 0 grams. However, if your simply simple weight loss stops, you must make changes. Until you attain your target weight, you remain in this phase.

As soon as you attain your desired weight, you enter this phase. Then you just continue easily eating this way for the rest of your life.

Chapter 17: Phases Of Atkins Diet

Atkins part one, additionally called Induction, is meant to jumpstart your simple weight loss. associate all-too-common idea is that part one of Atkins is that the whole program. In reality, it's the key to kick-starting your fat-easily burning metabolism. As you progress through the diet, you will notice the utmost grams of internet carbs you'll such consume whereas continued to slim, just keep your craving in restraint, and just keep alert and energized. this is often actually known as your carb balance. Phase one is all concerning dynamical the approach your body uses nutrients; thus, these initial few weeks are going to be essential to your simply simple weight loss journey. See details below on Induction and the way to urge started tojust gether with your low-carb diet. HOW LONG will part one LAST? The length of the Induction part depends on your simply simple weight loss goals. For some, part one maybe solely last fortnight. However, you'll safely follow it for much longer if you have got loads of simple weight to lose or opt to lose most of your excess pounds comparatively quickly. You will just keep during this part till you're fifteen pounds from your such good goal weight, thus Induction maybe not be necessary for those easily trying to lose less. to see if part one is true for you, look at our personalization tool or the compare simple plan page.

It is vital to starter motor your simply simple weight loss throughout the primary few weeks of a low-carb diet. That's why Atkins part one works by considerably shifting what you eat before sinking into a additional property way. jutting to the list of acceptable foods throughout part one can facilitate your body shift from easily burning primarily carbs to easily burning primarily fat. SUCH GOOD GOAL OF part ONE During Induction, it's vital to considerably drop your daily internet carb injust take to a median of twenty grams At this injust take level, nearly anyone begins to burn fat as their primary energy supply. The such good goal is to urge your body adjusted to the fat-easily burning method thus you will be able to slowly add additional carbs into your diet anon.

Southwest Chicken Soup By Andy

Ingredients

- 2 can (2 4 oz.) tomato (canned or chopped or stewed)
- 1 cup green leaves chilies
- 4 pound chicken breasts
- 2 cup sliced bell pepper 4 garlic cloves
- 2 sweet onion, tiny (chopped)
- 1 cup chicken broth
- 1/2 cup melted butter
- 2   chili seasoning blend simple using

Directions:

1. Easily cut the chicken breast into bits of your choice (bite-size).
2. In butter, sauté the bell pepper, garlic, and onion.
3. Add the chicken, red pepper, garlic, onions, and butter to the pan.
4. Easy cook the chicken just until it begins to shift color Preheat the crock pot and add the chicken stock, tomato, green chilies, and additional pan ingredients.
5. Add taco or chili spice to taste.
6. Set the crock pot on high for 1-5 minutes, then decrease to medium until ready to be served.
7. Garnish with sour cream and sharp cheddar.

Cheddar Cheese Soup

INGREDIENTS

- 2 tablespoon cornstarch (Atkins, ThickenThin not or Starch)
- 2 2 /2 cups heavy cream

- 8 ounces cheddar cheese, shredded (2 cups)
- 2 teaspoons paprika
- 2 /2 teaspoon salt
- 2 tablespoon unsalted butter
- 2 shallot, minced
- 2 2 /2 cups lower sodium vegetable broth

Directions:

1. Melt butter in a large saucepan over medium heat.

2. Add shallot and sauté until soft, about 4 minutes.
3. Add stock and bring to a simmer. Whisk in thickener; easy easy cook until mixture thickens, about 2 minutes.

4. Add cream and simmer, stirring occasionally, until hot.

5. Slowly whisk in cheese until melted and thoroughly combined.

6. Stir in paprika and salt and serve.

Chapter 1: The Truth About Free

Simply Simple Weight Loss Programs

The Internet gives various offers professing to be free just get-healthy simple plan however they're not generally as free as they guarantee to be.

Commonly, they are free preliminaries utilized as a secret to easily find out about their program. You ought to simple understand what you're searching for while looking with the expectation of complimentary assistance, so they don't easy turn out to be simply transitory free assistance.

The greatest tip to a program not being free is the point at which your Visa data is required, although they guarantee you will not be charged for utilizing the site. Frequently one more site will be connected on the first site and in some place in the fine print there will be a disclaimer alleging that you agree to the terms of the site by clicking certain options. Since they have your Mastercard on the document, you'll begin to see an unexplainable and repeasily eating charge until you have it dealt with either your bank or straightforwardly with the slippery site.

A few destinations have simple weight such reduction benefits that are free, and afterward, whenever you have joined, you'll see a proposal for complete admittance to their site for some measure of cash. The free piece of the site will ordinarily incorporate a rundown and clarification of activities as very well as certain recipes for low fat and low-calorie food sources. The total site will bait you in with individual consideration from a capable delegate to email or easy try and call you with basic encouragement. They maybe offer customized feast simple plan for yourself and exercise designs that will boost the viability of your exercise.

"Free preliminary" posted someplace on the site of a free just get-healthy plan is the clearest method for saying that it maybe be free for a time for testing. Mastercard data will in all likelihood be requested before you can just start the free preliminary, yet charges won't come until after the

time for testing is up. In some cases, these destinations will likewise offer an unconditional promise on the off chance that you're not happy with the program. Unexpectedly, it's typically a multi-day unconditional promise which isn't generally sufficient to show simple weight such reduction results as you could undoubtedly lose or simply put on simple weight because of same different variables in your day-to-day existence during that month!

There are programs accessible that are hoping to make the world a superior, better spot and are not hoping to just take your cash. These locales for the most part don't have an individual who will converse with you one-on-one yet they really do have networks of individuals very much like you attempting to shed pounds.

Gatherings are an incredible method for conveying these destinations and perceiving how others are doing on the program. Some of the time the locales will have the choices to easy allow you to tweak your dinner simple plan dependent on suppers they had proactively assembled. Messages loaded with sound tips are likewise sent from the free just get-healthy plans, so when

you easily find the one you actually need
be prepared for a better way of life.

Protein Packed Almond Pancakes

With Blueberries

Ingredients:

- 1 an ounce of cottage cheese
- 2 tablespoons of Whey protein, vanilla Flavored
- 1/2 cup of blueberries, fresh
- 2 /2 6 cup of flour, almond blanched
- ¾ of a whole egg, large
- 2 /8 cup of flour, whole grain soy
- 1/2 teaspoons of baker's style baking powder

Direction:

1. First, combine your two flours, baking powder, and protein powder, until thoroughly mixed.
2. Add in your fresh egg and cottage cheese and stir to blend thoroughly.
3. Then, heat the oil at medium heat in a large skillet.
4. Add some canola oil.
5. When your skillet is hot enough, add at least 1/2 cup of your pancake batter and boil until the bubbles form.
6. Easy cook until firm to the touch after flipping.
7. Serve with a garnish of your fresh blueberries and enjoy.

Apple Muffins With A Pecan And Cinnamon Streusel

Ingredients:

- 2 2/4 cups of almond flour
- 1 cup of pecans, easily cut into halves
- 10 teaspoons of cinnamon, ground
- 2 /4 teaspoons of salt
- 24 teaspoons of sugar substitute
- Dash of stevia
- 2 tablespoons of butter, unsalted
- 2 fresh eggs, large
- ½ cup of coconut milk, unsweetened
- 2 teaspoons of pure vanilla
- 2 tablespoons of coconut flour
- 2 teaspoon of baker's style baking powder
- 2/4 cup of apple, chopped

Direction:

1. Heat the oven to 450 degrees. Line a cupcake pan with cupcake paper liners while the oven is heasily eating up.
2. Add the almond flour, chopped pecans, two tablespoons of ground cinnamon, salt, sugar substitute, dashes of stevia, and melted butter to a small bowl. Stir very well to mix until crumbly. Set aside.
3. Then add the fresh eggs, coconut milk, pure vanilla, remaining sugar substitute, dashes of stevia, and ground cinnamon to a large bowl. Stir very well to mix.
4. Add one cup of almond flour, coconut flour, a dash of salt, baking powder, and chopped apples. Stir very well to mix.
5. Pour the batter among the muffin cups into the pan.

6. Top off with two tablespoons of the streusel.
7. Place into the oven to bake for 30 to 35 minutes.
8. Remove and easy allow to sit for 30 to 35 minutes before serving.

Sheet Pan Shrimp Fajitas

Ingredients:

- 2 teaspoons plus 2 /4 cup canola oil, divided
- 2 garlic cloves
- 2 teaspoon kosher salt
- • 1 teaspoon dried oregano
- • 1 teaspoon chili powder
- • 1 teaspoon sweet paprika
- • 1 teaspoon cayenne pepper
- • 1/2 teaspoon ground cumin
- 2 pound (42 /6 0 size) raw shrimp, de-veined and shelled
- 6 flour tortillas
- Mexican crema, sour cream, or Greek yogurt
- 2 limes
- 2   red bell pepper, seeded and julienned

- • 1 green bell pepper, seeded and julienned
- • 1 large yellow onion, thinly sliced

Direction:

1. 2 . Preheat the oven to 450°F. Set the sheet pan close by.
2. Juice 2 1 of the limes. Easily cut the other lime half into six wedges and set them aside.
3. 4 . Toss the bell peppers and onion into the 2 teaspoons of canola oil until coated.
4. Scatter them onto the sheet pan in a single layer.
5. Pour the lime juice and garlic into a blender, adding in the remaining oil in a steady stream.
6. Add the salt and spices, pulsing once to combine.

7. Marinate the shrimp, tossing to coat in a large zip-seal bag for 20 to 25 minutes.
8. Meanwhile, roast the bell pepper and onion for 2 0 minutes.
9. Remove the shrimp from the marinade.
10. Polka dot the shrimp onto the sheet pan of roasted veggies.
11. Roast for 8 minutes more or until pink and fragrant.
12. Heat some flour tortillas and set out the Mexican crema or sour cream to serve with the lime wedges.

Broiled Lobster

Ingredients:
- 2 tablespoons butter stick, unsalted, melted
- 4 lbs. Lobster
- Salt to taste
- 2 teaspoon minced garlic
- 1/2 cup olive oil

Direction:

1. Heat the rack by placing it 6 inches away from the broiler flame.
2. Mix the melted butter, olive oil, and garlic. Just keep the mixture warm.
3. Easily cut the lobster in half, crack its claws and scoop the viscera out. Remove the green sacs.
4. Place them on broiling pans with the easily cut side up.
5. With the butter mixture, brush the lobsters and season them with salt.

6. Brush with the mixture after 4 minutes and broil for 5 to 10 minutes.
7. Serve one lobster to each guest.

Belgian Waffles Recipe

Easy cook Ingredients

- 1 teaspoon salt & 1/2 cup Heavy Cream
- 4 large Fresh eggs & 2 tablespoon Sugar-Free Syrup
- 1/2 cup Water
- 4 tablespoons Sucralose Based Sweetener
- 2 cup Whole Grain Soy Flour & 4 teaspoons Baking Powder

1. Warmth waffle iron per aker's guidelines. Whisk tojust gether soy flour, sugar substitute, preparing powder and salt.
2. Just include cream, fresh eggs and syrup and mix until very much mixed. Just include cold water 2 tablespoon at once until hitter is effectively

spoonable and spreadable, about the consistency of a thick hotcake batter.

3. Shower waffle iron with oil splash.

4. Spot around 4 tablespoons of hitter in the focal point of a waffle iron.

5. Easy cook as indicated by producer's directions until fresh and dim brilliant darker.

6. Rehash with the rest of the batter. Serve warm.

Garlic Roasted Cauliflower

Ingredients:

- 1/2 cup olive oil
- 10 garlic cloves, crushed and minced
- 4 cups chopped cauliflower florets
- 2 teaspoon ground black pepper
- 2 teaspoon kosher salt
- 2 tablespoon parsley

Directions:

1. Preheat oven to 450 degrees Fahrenheit.
2. Combine the cauliflower with salt and pepper, parsley, garlic and oil in a bowl. Toss well.
3. Pour the mixture into a jellyroll pan.
4. Simply put in the oven and bake for 46 minutes or up to an hour.

5. Just take it out of the oven every 2 6 minutes to stir.
6. *Store leftovers in an airtight container inside the fridge.
7. Reheat in the microwave on high for 1-5 minutes.

General Wong's Beef And Broccoli

Ingredients:

- 2 pound of steak, easily cut into strips
  - 2 pound of stemmed and cleaved into florets broccoli
  - 2 /4 cup of shellfish sauce
  - 2 /4 cup of sherry
  - 2 tablespoon of minced ginger
  - 2 tablespoon of minced garlic
  - 2 tablespoon of olive oil
  - 2 tablespoon of soy sauce
  - 2 tablespoon of sesame oil
  - 2 teaspoon of cornstarch

Direction:

1. Simple using a bowl, add the clam sauce, sherry, minced ginger, minced garlic, olive oil, soy sauce, sesame oil, cornstarch and mix it until it is appropriately blended.
2. Then, at that point, add the steak, broccoli, cover it very well and permit it to marinate for 35 to 40 minutes or overnight.

3. Then preheat your air fryer to 450degrees Fahrenheit.

4. After marinating, place the marinade steak and broccoli in your air fryer.

5. Easy cook it for 2 6 minutes at a 450degrees Fahrenheit or until it is done.

6. Serve and appreciate alongside the white rice!

Braised Leeks And Fennel

Ingredients:

.

- 4 leeks, diced
    - .2 fennel bulb,
    - .diced 2 cup
    - .chiken   broth
  Pinch pepper
- .

- 4 Tbsp unsalted butter
    - .2 Tbsp fresh lemon juice

- ⅓ cup parsley, chopped

Directions:

1. Preheat stove to 450 F
2. In a 2 2 x 10 glass baking dish, add the leeks, fennel.

2. Pour in the chicken stock. Season with pepper.

3. Easily cut up spread.

4. Place over the fixings. Cover baking dish with aluminum foil.
4. Bake 25 to 30 minutes.

5. Eliminate from oven.
6 . Stir in lemon juice. Decorate with parsley. Serve.

Seafood Risotto

Ingredients

- Chopped parsley to taste
- 6 tablespoons of some extra virgin olive oil
- 2 cloves of garlic, 2 shallots
- Green pepper to taste Salt to taste.
- 2 lt. of vejust getable broth approx
- 4 20 g. of Rice
- 450gr. of clean mussels
- 450gr. of clean clams
- 2 glass of white wine
- 550 gr. of Calamari
- 4 shelled prawns
- 250gr. of peeled prawns

some extra

Direction:

1. Simply put the cleaned mussels and clams in a non-stick pan tojust gether with 2 tablespoons of some extra virgin olive oil and 2 clove of peeled garlic.
2. Let them open on a high flame. Then drain and peel them, just keeping some with their shells aside to garnish the dish.
3. Easy turn on the heat and reduce their easily cooking juices.
4. Filter it and just keep it aside. Pour 4 tablespoons of some extra virgin olive oil into a non-stick pan and add the peeled and thinly sliced shallots and 2 whole peeled clove of garlic. Let it dry and then add the rice.
5. Toast it for a couple of minutes and pour in the white wine.

6. Let the wine evaporate over a high flame and add the clean squid that you have previously washed very well under fresh running water, then easily cut the bags into

7. washers and the tentacles into small pieces.
8. Immediately pour the easily cooking juices of the seafood kept aside.
9. Stir, let the rice absorb the seafood sauce, and then start adding a ladle of boiling vejust getable broth.
10.   Just continue easily cooking the rice for 20 to 25   minutes, adding more broth when the previous one has been absorbed.
11.   When the rice is cooked for a few minutes, add the prawns and shrimps and mix.
12.   After a couple of minutes, add the mussels and shelled clams.

13. Stir, aleasy way gently, and let the easily cooking liquid absorb almost completely.

14. Easy turn off the heat and distribute the risotto in individual bowls.

15. Garnish with shellfish complete with shell and sprinkle with a light grind of green pepper and chopped fresh parsley.

16. Serve your seafood risotto immediately hot and enjoy your meal!

Bowl Of Berries

4 individuals Ingredients:
• 1 cup of strawberries
 • 1 lime juice
 • 1/2 cup of new basil, finely hacked • 1 cup of raspberries
 • 1 cup of blueberries

Directions:

1. Remove originates from berries and cleave them in a bowl.

2. Mix lemon juice with berries. 4 . Topping with slashed basil, and it's prepared to serve.

3. Serve this heavenly formula.

Parmesan Green Salad

Ingredients:

- 2 cup almond milk
- 2 half of cups ice cubes
- 2 cups spinach
- 2 packet Stevia
- 1/2 cup vanilla protein powder
- 1 avocado, pitted and chopped

Directions:
1. Pour milk in the blender.
2. Add the spinach and the relaxation of the ingredients.
3. Blend on excessive till smooth.